SMOOTHIES FOR COLITIS

DR. MAUREEN MOORE

TABLE OF CONTENT

CHAPTER ONE

Introduction

Certainly! Smoothies can be a convenient and nutritious option for individuals with colitis, as they provide a way to incorporate essential nutrients without causing irritation to the digestive tract.

Colitis, including conditions like ulcerative colitis and Crohn's disease, involves inflammation of the colon, and certain dietary choices can help manage symptoms. Here's a comprehensive introduction to smoothies for colitis

Principles for Colitis-Friendly Smoothies:

Blended Consistency: Opt for smoothies with a well-blended and homogeneous consistency to reduce the mechanical work of digestion.

Low-Fiber Choices: Choose fruits and vegetables that are low in insoluble fiber to minimize potential irritation to the digestive tract.

Nutrient Density: Aim for nutrient-dense smoothies that provide a variety of essential vitamins and minerals without overwhelming the digestive system.

Balanced Macronutrients: Include a balance of carbohydrates, proteins, and healthy fats to support overall nutritional needs.

Hydration Emphasis: Incorporate ingredients with high water content to help maintain hydration levels.

Mindful Sweetening: Be mindful of sweeteners, opting for natural sources like honey or maple syrup in moderation, and minimizing added sugars.

Easy-to-Digest Proteins: Choose proteins that are easy to digest, such as protein powder, Greek yogurt, or silken tofu.

Lactose Considerations: If using dairy, opt for lactose-free options or consider non-dairy alternatives like almond or coconut milk.

Probiotic Inclusion (if tolerated): Some individuals find probiotics beneficial. Consider including yogurt with live cultures or a probiotic supplement, but consult with healthcare providers first.

Tips for Making Colitis-Friendly Smoothies:

Choose Low-Fiber Fruits and Vegetables: Opt for fruits and vegetables that are lower in insoluble fiber to minimize irritation. Examples include bananas, peeled and cooked apples, and peeled cucumbers.

Include Healthy Fats: Add sources of healthy fats like avocados, nut butters, or seeds for added calories and nutritional density.

Use Lactose-Free Dairy or Alternatives: If you include dairy, choose lactose-free options or consider non-dairy alternatives like almond or coconut milk.

Avoid High-Sugar Additions: Minimize added sugars, as excessive sugar intake can contribute to inflammation. Sweeten your smoothie with natural options like honey or maple syrup in moderation.

Experiment with Probiotics: Some individuals find probiotics beneficial. Consider adding yogurt with live cultures or a probiotic supplement, but check with your healthcare provider first.

Include Easily Digestible Proteins: Choose easily digestible protein sources, such as protein powder, Greek yogurt, or silken tofu.

Important Considerations:

Individual Variability: Colitis affects individuals differently, so it's essential to monitor how your body responds to different ingredients.

Consult with Healthcare Professionals: Before making significant dietary changes, consult with your healthcare provider or a registered dietitian who can provide personalized guidance based on your specific condition.

Gradual Introductions: Introduce new ingredients gradually to identify any potential triggers or intolerances.

Remember, dietary recommendations can vary, and it's crucial to tailor your choices to your specific needs and preferences. Always consult with your healthcare team for personalized advice on managing colitis through diet.

Benefits of Smoothies for Colitis

Smoothies can offer several potential benefits for individuals with colitis. It's important to note that the impact of smoothies can vary from person to person, and it's essential to pay attention to individual responses. Here are some potential benefits of incorporating smoothies into the diet for individuals with colitis:

Easy Digestibility: The blending process breaks down food into a more digestible form, reducing the mechanical work required by the digestive system. This can be particularly beneficial for individuals with colitis who may experience difficulty digesting certain foods.

Nutrient Density: Smoothies allow for the incorporation of a variety of nutrient-dense ingredients, providing essential vitamins, minerals, and antioxidants. This can contribute to overall nutrition and support the body's healing processes.

Hydration Support: Many smoothie ingredients, such as fruits and vegetables, have high water content, contributing to hydration. Maintaining adequate hydration is crucial for individuals with colitis, as dehydration can exacerbate symptoms.

Balanced Nutrition: Smoothies can be customized to include a balance of macronutrients (carbohydrates, proteins, and healthy fats). This balance supports sustained energy levels and helps meet nutritional needs.

Anti-Inflammatory Ingredients: Ingredients with anti-inflammatory properties, such as ginger, turmeric, and certain fruits, can be included in smoothies to potentially help manage inflammation associated with colitis.

Probiotic Inclusion: Some smoothie ingredients, like yogurt with live cultures or kefir, can introduce beneficial probiotics to support gut health. Probiotics may contribute to a balanced gut microbiome, potentially aiding in symptom management.

Individualized Ingredient Selection: Smoothies offer flexibility in ingredient selection, allowing individuals to tailor recipes to their specific tolerances and preferences. This customization can help avoid trigger foods and accommodate individual dietary needs.

Meal Replacement Option: Smoothies can serve as a convenient and easily digestible meal replacement, providing essential nutrients during periods when solid foods may be challenging to consume.

Gradual Introduction of Ingredients: Individuals with colitis often need to be cautious about introducing new foods. Smoothies allow for the gradual introduction of ingredients, making it easier to identify and manage any potential triggers.

Texture Modification: Blending allows for texture modification, making it possible to create smoother consistencies that are gentler on the digestive tract. This can be particularly helpful for those with sensitivity to rough or fibrous textures.

It's important to emphasize that while smoothies can offer these potential benefits, individual responses may vary.

Some individuals may find certain ingredients more tolerable than others, and it's advisable to consult with healthcare professionals or a registered dietitian for personalized guidance tailored to specific needs and preferences. Regular communication with healthcare providers is essential for effective management of colitis through dietary choices.

Causes of Colitis

Colitis refers to inflammation of the colon (large intestine), and there are various causes for this condition. The specific cause can help determine the type of colitis a person has. Here are some common causes of colitis:

Inflammatory Bowel Disease (IBD): a. Ulcerative Colitis: This is a chronic condition characterized by inflammation and ulcers in the lining of the colon and rectum.

b. Crohn's Disease: Another form of IBD that can affect any part of the digestive tract, including the colon. It often involves deep inflammation and can lead to complications.

Infection: Bacterial, viral, or parasitic infections can cause infectious colitis. Common culprits include E. coli, Salmonella, Shigella, Campylobacter, and Clostridium difficile (C. difficile).

Ischemic Colitis: Reduced blood flow to the colon due to blood vessel blockages or other vascular issues can lead to ischemic colitis. This can result in inflammation and damage to the colon.

Microscopic Colitis: This type of colitis is characterized by chronic, watery diarrhea and inflammation that is visible only under a microscope. The exact cause is unclear, but it's often associated with autoimmune factors.

Radiation Colitis: Exposure to radiation, often used in cancer treatment, can lead to inflammation and damage to the colon, resulting in radiation colitis.

Autoimmune Reactions: Some forms of colitis may result from autoimmune reactions, where the immune system mistakenly attacks the cells of the colon. Examples include collagenous colitis and lymphocytic colitis.

Allergic Reactions: Colitis can sometimes be triggered by allergic reactions to certain foods or substances, leading to inflammation in the colon.

Diverticulitis: Inflammation of small pouches (diverticula) that can form in the walls of the colon, known as diverticulitis, can cause colitis-like symptoms.

Medication-Induced Colitis: Certain medications, such as nonsteroidal anti-inflammatory drugs (NSAIDs), antibiotics, and some anti-hypertensive drugs, may cause colitis as a side effect.

Chemical Colitis: Exposure to certain chemicals, such as harsh cleaning agents or toxic substances, can lead to inflammation in the colon.

It's important to note that the specific cause of colitis can vary among individuals, and in some cases, the exact cause may not be clearly identified.

Additionally, a combination of genetic, environmental, and immune system factors may contribute to the development of colitis in some individuals. Proper diagnosis and treatment are crucial, and individuals experiencing symptoms of colitis should seek medical attention for a thorough evaluation and appropriate management.

Symptoms of Colitis

Colitis is characterized by inflammation of the colon, and the symptoms can vary depending on the specific type and underlying cause of the condition. Common symptoms of colitis may include:

Abdominal Pain: Persistent or intermittent abdominal pain and discomfort, often crampy in nature, can be a prominent symptom of colitis.

Diarrhea: Frequent bowel movements with loose or watery stools are a hallmark symptom of colitis. In some cases, blood or mucus may be present in the stool.

Rectal Bleeding: Blood in the stool or visible rectal bleeding may occur, especially in conditions like ulcerative colitis.

Urgency to Defecate: A sense of urgency to have a bowel movement is common, and individuals may feel the need to rush to the restroom.

Weight Loss: Unexplained weight loss may occur due to a combination of factors, including decreased appetite and nutrient malabsorption.

Fatigue: Chronic inflammation and the body's response to it can lead to fatigue and a general feeling of weakness.

Fever: Inflammatory processes can sometimes result in an elevated body temperature, leading to fever.

Nausea and Vomiting: Some individuals with colitis may experience nausea and vomiting, especially during flare-ups or periods of active inflammation.

Incomplete Bowel Movements: Feeling of incomplete evacuation after a bowel movement can be a symptom of colitis.

Joint Pain: Inflammatory bowel diseases, like Crohn's disease and ulcerative colitis, can be associated with joint pain and inflammation.

Skin Problems: Skin issues, such as rashes or sores, may occur in some individuals with colitis, particularly in autoimmune forms of the disease.

Changes in Bowel Habits: Colitis can cause alterations in bowel habits, including constipation in some cases.

It's important to note that the severity and combination of symptoms can vary widely among individuals. Additionally, symptoms may come and go, with periods of remission and flare-ups. If you are experiencing symptoms suggestive of colitis, it's crucial to seek medical attention promptly.

A healthcare professional can conduct a thorough evaluation, which may involve physical examinations, laboratory tests, imaging studies, and endoscopic procedures, to determine the underlying cause and guide appropriate treatment. Early diagnosis and management are key to improving the quality of life for individuals with colitis.

CHAPTER TWO

1. Banana Berry Soothing Smoothie

Ingredients:

1 ripe banana

1/2 cup fresh blueberries

1/2 cup strawberries, hulled

1/2 cup plain Greek yogurt

1 tablespoon honey (optional)

1 cup cold chamomile tea (brewed and chilled)

Ice cubes

Instructions:

In a blender, combine the banana, blueberries, strawberries, Greek yogurt, and honey.

Add chamomile tea to achieve the desired consistency.

Blend until smooth.

Add ice cubes and blend again.

Pour into a glass and enjoy immediately.

Cooking Time: Approximately 5 minutes

2. Papaya and Ginger Digestive Smoothie

Ingredients:

1 cup ripe papaya, diced

1/2 inch fresh ginger, peeled and grated

1/2 cup coconut water

1 tablespoon chia seeds

1 tablespoon flaxseed meal

1/2 teaspoon turmeric (optional)

Ice cubes

Instructions:

Combine papaya, ginger, coconut water, chia seeds, flaxseed meal, and turmeric (if using) in a blender.

Blend until smooth.

Add ice cubes and blend again.

Pour into a glass and serve immediately.

Cooking Time: Approximately 5 minutes

3. Spinach and Pineapple Anti-Inflammatory Smoothie

Ingredients:

1 cup fresh pineapple chunks

1 cup fresh spinach leaves

1/2 cucumber, peeled and sliced

1 tablespoon fresh mint leaves

1 tablespoon hemp seeds

1 cup coconut water

Ice cubes

Instructions:

In a blender, combine pineapple chunks, spinach, cucumber, mint leaves, and hemp seeds.

Add coconut water to achieve the desired consistency.

Blend until smooth.

Add ice cubes and blend again.

Pour into a glass and enjoy.

Cooking Time: Approximately 5 minutes

4. Coconut Blueberry Bliss Smoothie

Ingredients:

1/2 cup frozen blueberries

1/2 cup coconut milk (unsweetened)

1/2 cup plain lactose-free yogurt

1 tablespoon chia seeds

1 tablespoon honey (optional)

Ice cubes

Instructions:

Blend blueberries, coconut milk, lactose-free yogurt, chia seeds, and honey until smooth.

Add ice cubes and blend again.

Pour into a glass and enjoy.

Cooking Time: Approximately 5 minutes

5. Aloe Vera Green Smoothie

Ingredients:

1 cup fresh spinach leaves

1/2 cucumber, peeled and sliced

1/2 cup pineapple chunks

2 tablespoons aloe vera gel

1 tablespoon fresh lime juice

1 cup coconut water

Ice cubes

Instructions:

Blend spinach, cucumber, pineapple, aloe vera gel, lime juice, and coconut water until smooth.

Add ice cubes and blend again.

Pour into a glass and serve immediately.

Cooking Time: Approximately 5 minutes

6. Peach Ginger Delight Smoothie

Ingredients:

1 cup ripe peaches, diced

1/2 teaspoon fresh ginger, grated

1/2 cup almond milk (unsweetened)

1 tablespoon flaxseed meal

1 tablespoon almond butter

Ice cubes

Instructions:

Combine peaches, ginger, almond milk, flaxseed meal, and almond butter in a blender.

Blend until smooth.

Add ice cubes and blend again.

Pour into a glass and enjoy.

Cooking Time: Approximately 5 minutes

7. Carrot Cake Smoothie

Ingredients:

1 cup carrots, chopped

1/2 cup unsweetened applesauce

1/4 cup rolled oats

1/2 teaspoon ground cinnamon

1/4 teaspoon nutmeg

1 cup almond milk (unsweetened)

Ice cubes

Instructions:

Blend carrots, applesauce, oats, cinnamon, nutmeg, and almond milk until smooth.

Add ice cubes and blend again.

Pour into a glass and savor the carrot cake flavor.

Cooking Time: Approximately 5 minutes

8. Mango Mint Refresh Smoothie

Ingredients:

1 cup fresh mango chunks

1/4 cup fresh mint leaves

1/2 cup coconut water

1/2 cup plain Greek yogurt

1 tablespoon chia seeds

Ice cubes

Instructions:

Blend mango chunks, mint leaves, coconut water, Greek yogurt, and chia seeds until smooth.

Add ice cubes and blend again.

Pour into a glass and enjoy the refreshing taste.

Cooking Time: Approximately 5 minutes

9. Kiwi Kiwi Digestive Boost Smoothie

Ingredients:

2 kiwis, peeled and sliced

1/2 cup pineapple chunks

1/2 cup spinach leaves

1 tablespoon fresh lime juice

1 tablespoon honey (optional)

1 cup coconut water

Ice cubes

Instructions:

Blend kiwis, pineapple, spinach, lime juice, honey, and coconut water until smooth.

Add ice cubes and blend again.

Pour into a glass and relish the digestive boost.

Cooking Time: Approximately 5 minutes

10. Cantaloupe and Mint Cooler Smoothie

Ingredients:

1 cup cantaloupe, diced

1/4 cup fresh mint leaves

1/2 cup watermelon, diced

1/2 cup cucumber, peeled and sliced

1 tablespoon chia seeds

1 cup coconut water

Ice cubes

Instructions:

Blend cantaloupe, mint leaves, watermelon, cucumber, chia seeds, and coconut water until smooth.

Add ice cubes and blend again.

Pour into a glass and enjoy the refreshing cooler.

Cooking Time: Approximately 5 minutes

11. Pineapple Turmeric Soother Smoothie

Ingredients:

1 cup pineapple chunks

1/2 teaspoon ground turmeric

1/2 cup plain Greek yogurt

1 tablespoon honey (optional)

1/2 cup almond milk (unsweetened)

Ice cubes

Instructions:

Combine pineapple, turmeric, Greek yogurt, honey, and almond milk in a blender.

Blend until smooth.

Add ice cubes and blend again.

Pour into a glass and soothe your senses.

Cooking Time: Approximately 5 minutes

12. Blueberry Basil Bliss Smoothie

Ingredients:

1/2 cup frozen blueberries

1/2 cup fresh basil leaves

1/2 cup cucumber, peeled and sliced

1 tablespoon chia seeds

1 cup coconut water

Ice cubes

Instructions:

Blend blueberries, basil leaves, cucumber, chia seeds, and coconut water until smooth.

Add ice cubes and blend again.

Pour into a glass and relish the unique flavor.

Cooking Time: Approximately 5 minutes

13. Cherry Almond Indulgence Smoothie

Ingredients:

1 cup frozen cherries

1/4 cup almonds

1/2 cup almond milk (unsweetened)

1/2 cup plain lactose-free yogurt

1 tablespoon honey (optional)

Ice cubes

Instructions:

Blend cherries, almonds, almond milk, lactose-free yogurt, and honey until smooth.

Add ice cubes and blend again.

Pour into a glass and indulge in the cherry-almond delight.

Cooking Time:

Approximately 5 minutes

14. Pear Ginger Elixir Smoothie

Ingredients:

1 ripe pear, diced

1/2 teaspoon fresh ginger, grated

1/2 cup coconut water

1/2 cup plain Greek yogurt

1 tablespoon chia seeds

Ice cubes

Instructions:

Blend pear, ginger, coconut water, Greek yogurt, and chia seeds until smooth.

Add ice cubes and blend again.

Pour into a glass and savor the pear-ginger elixir.

Cooking Time:

Approximately 5 minutes

15. Raspberry Avocado Delight Smoothie

Ingredients:

1/2 cup frozen raspberries

1/2 avocado, peeled and diced

1/2 cup spinach leaves

1 tablespoon flaxseed meal

1 cup almond milk (unsweetened)

Ice cubes

Instructions:

Combine raspberries, avocado, spinach, flaxseed meal, and almond milk in a blender.

Blend until smooth.

Add ice cubes and blend again.

Pour into a glass and enjoy the delightful combination.

Cooking Time: Approximately 5 minutes

16. Minty Melon Medley Smoothie

Ingredients:

1 cup honeydew melon, diced

1/2 cup cantaloupe, diced

1/4 cup fresh mint leaves

1/2 cup coconut water

1/2 cup plain lactose-free yogurt

Ice cubes

Instructions:

Blend honeydew melon, cantaloupe, mint leaves, coconut water, and lactose-free yogurt until smooth.

Add ice cubes and blend again.

Pour into a glass and revel in the minty melon medley.

Cooking Time: Approximately 5 minutes

17. Strawberry Basil Infusion Smoothie

Ingredients:

1 cup fresh strawberries, hulled

1/4 cup fresh basil leaves

1/2 cup cucumber, peeled and sliced

1 tablespoon chia seeds

1 cup coconut water

Ice cubes

Instructions:

Blend strawberries, basil leaves, cucumber, chia seeds, and coconut water until smooth.

Add ice cubes and blend again.

Pour into a glass and indulge in the strawberry-basil infusion.

Cooking Time: Approximately 5 minutes

18. Pomegranate Citrus Splash Smoothie

Ingredients:

1/2 cup pomegranate seeds

Juice of 1 orange

Juice of 1 grapefruit

1/2 cup plain Greek yogurt

1 tablespoon honey (optional)

Ice cubes

Instructions:

Blend pomegranate seeds, orange juice, grapefruit juice, Greek yogurt, and honey until smooth.

Add ice cubes and blend again.

Pour into a glass and enjoy the refreshing citrus splash.

Cooking Time: Approximately 5 minutes

19. Cucumber Celery Green Goddess Smoothie

Ingredients:

1/2 cucumber, peeled and sliced

2 celery stalks, chopped

1/2 cup pineapple chunks

1 tablespoon fresh lime juice

1 tablespoon chia seeds

1 cup coconut water

Ice cubes

Instructions:

Combine cucumber, celery, pineapple, lime juice, chia seeds, and coconut water in a blender.

Blend until smooth.

Add ice cubes and blend again.

Pour into a glass and relish the green goddess goodness.

Cooking Time: Approximately 5 minutes

20. Fig and Banana Smoothie

Ingredients:

2 ripe bananas

4 fresh figs, stemmed and halved

1/2 cup almond milk (unsweetened)

1 tablespoon almond butter

1 tablespoon chia seeds

Ice cubes

Instructions:

Blend bananas, figs, almond milk, almond butter, and chia seeds until smooth.

Add ice cubes and blend again.

Pour into a glass and savor the sweet combination of fig and banana.

Cooking Time: Approximately 5 minutes

21. Turmeric Mango Tango Smoothie

Ingredients:

1 cup mango chunks

1/2 teaspoon ground turmeric

1/2 cup coconut water

1/2 cup plain Greek yogurt

1 tablespoon chia seeds

Ice cubes

Instructions:

Blend mango chunks, turmeric, Greek yogurt, chia seeds, and coconut water until smooth.

Add ice cubes and blend again.

Pour into a glass and enjoy the tropical turmeric twist.

Cooking Time: Approximately 5 minutes

22. Lemon Raspberry Zest Smoothie

Ingredients:

1 cup fresh raspberries

Juice of 1 lemon

1/2 cup plain lactose-free yogurt

1 tablespoon flaxseed meal

1 tablespoon honey (optional)

Ice cubes

Instructions:

Combine raspberries, lemon juice, lactose-free yogurt, flaxseed meal, and honey in a blender.

Blend until smooth.

Add ice cubes and blend again.

Pour into a glass and savor the zesty goodness.

Cooking Time: Approximately 5 minutes

23. Orange Carrot Crush Smoothie

Ingredients:

1 cup carrots, chopped

Juice of 2 oranges

1/2 cup almond milk (unsweetened)

1 tablespoon fresh ginger, grated

1 tablespoon chia seeds

Ice cubes

Instructions:

Blend carrots, orange juice, almond milk, ginger, and chia seeds until smooth.

Add ice cubes and blend again.

Pour into a glass and crush the orange-carrot combination.

Cooking Time: Approximately 5 minutes

24. Pumpkin Pie Protein Smoothie

Ingredients:

1/2 cup canned pumpkin puree

1/2 teaspoon pumpkin spice

1/2 cup plain Greek yogurt

1/4 cup rolled oats

1 tablespoon almond butter

1 cup almond milk (unsweetened)

Ice cubes

Instructions:

Blend pumpkin puree, pumpkin spice, Greek yogurt, rolled oats, almond butter, and almond milk until smooth.

Add ice cubes and blend again.

Pour into a glass and enjoy the pumpkin pie protein goodness.

Cooking Time: Approximately 5 minutes

25. Blackberry Basil Bliss Smoothie

Ingredients:

1/2 cup fresh blackberries

1/4 cup fresh basil leaves

1/2 cup cucumber, peeled and sliced

1 tablespoon chia seeds

1 cup coconut water

Ice cubes

Instructions:

Blend blackberries, basil leaves, cucumber, chia seeds, and coconut water until smooth.

Add ice cubes and blend again.

Pour into a glass and relish the unique blackberry-basil bliss.

Cooking Time: Approximately 5 minutes

26. Mint Chocolate Chip Delight Smoothie

Ingredients:

1 cup fresh spinach leaves

1/2 teaspoon peppermint extract

1 tablespoon cacao nibs

1/2 cup plain lactose-free yogurt

1 tablespoon honey (optional)

1 cup almond milk (unsweetened)

Ice cubes

Instructions:

Blend spinach, peppermint extract, cacao nibs, lactose-free yogurt, honey, and almond milk until smooth.

Add ice cubes and blend again.

Pour into a glass and delight in the mint chocolate chip goodness.

Cooking Time: Approximately 5 minutes

27. Chia Berry Protein Boost Smoothie

Ingredients:

1/2 cup mixed berries (strawberries, blueberries, raspberries)

1 tablespoon chia seeds

1/2 cup plain Greek yogurt

1 scoop protein powder (unflavored)

1 tablespoon honey (optional)

1 cup almond milk (unsweetened)

Ice cubes

Instructions:

Blend mixed berries, chia seeds, Greek yogurt, protein powder, honey, and almond milk until smooth.

Add ice cubes and blend again.

Pour into a glass and enjoy the protein-packed berry boost.

Cooking Time: Approximately 5 minutes

28. Peach Basil Fusion Smoothie

Ingredients:

1 cup ripe peaches, diced

1/4 cup fresh basil leaves

1/2 cup plain lactose-free yogurt

1 tablespoon flaxseed meal

1 tablespoon honey (optional)

1 cup coconut water

Ice cubes

Instructions:

Combine peaches, basil leaves, lactose-free yogurt, flaxseed meal, honey, and coconut water in a blender.

Blend until smooth.

Add ice cubes and blend again.

Pour into a glass and savor the peach-basil fusion.

Cooking Time: Approximately 5 minutes

29. Vanilla Almond Comfort Smoothie

Ingredients:

1/2 teaspoon vanilla extract

1/4 cup almonds

1/2 cup plain Greek yogurt

1 tablespoon chia seeds

1 tablespoon honey (optional)

1 cup almond milk (unsweetened)

Ice cubes

Instructions:

Blend vanilla extract, almonds, Greek yogurt, chia seeds, honey, and almond milk until smooth.

Add ice cubes and blend again.

Pour into a glass and find comfort in the vanilla almond goodness.

Cooking Time: Approximately 5 minutes

30. Blueberry Basil Detox Smoothie

Ingredients:

1/2 cup frozen blueberries

1/4 cup fresh basil leaves

1/2 cucumber, peeled and sliced

Juice of 1 lemon

1 tablespoon chia seeds

1 cup coconut water

Ice cubes

Instructions:

Blend blueberries, basil leaves, cucumber, lemon juice, chia seeds, and coconut water until smooth.

Add ice cubes and blend again.

Pour into a glass and detox with the blueberry-basil blend.

Cooking Time: Approximately 5 minutes

31. Raspberry Coconut Euphoria Smoothie

Ingredients:

1/2 cup fresh raspberries

1/2 cup coconut milk (unsweetened)

1/2 cup plain Greek yogurt

1 tablespoon flaxseed meal

1 tablespoon honey (optional)

Ice cubes

Instructions:

Blend raspberries, coconut milk, Greek yogurt, flaxseed meal, and honey until smooth.

Add ice cubes and blend again.

Pour into a glass and experience the raspberry-coconut euphoria.

Cooking Time: Approximately 5 minutes

32. Green Tea Berry Burst Smoothie

Ingredients:

1 green tea bag (brewed and chilled)

1/2 cup mixed berries (strawberries, blueberries, raspberries)

1/2 cup plain lactose-free yogurt

1 tablespoon chia seeds

1 tablespoon honey (optional)

Ice cubes

Instructions:

Brew green tea and let it chill.

In a blender, combine chilled green tea, mixed berries, lactose-free yogurt, chia seeds, and honey.

Blend until smooth.

Add ice cubes and blend again.

Pour into a glass and enjoy the green tea berry burst.

Cooking Time: Approximately 5 minutes

33. Mango Basil Breeze Smoothie

Ingredients:

1 cup mango chunks

1/4 cup fresh basil leaves

1/2 cup plain Greek yogurt

1 tablespoon chia seeds

1 tablespoon honey (optional)

1 cup coconut water

Ice cubes

Instructions:

Blend mango chunks, basil leaves, Greek yogurt, chia seeds, honey, and coconut water until smooth.

Add ice cubes and blend again.

Pour into a glass and enjoy the mango-basil breeze.

Cooking Time: Approximately 5 minutes

34. Cranberry Orange Zing Smoothie

Ingredients:

1/2 cup cranberries (fresh or frozen)

Juice of 1 orange

1/2 cup plain lactose-free yogurt

1 tablespoon flaxseed meal

1 tablespoon honey (optional)

1 cup almond milk (unsweetened)

Ice cubes

Instructions:

Blend cranberries, orange juice, lactose-free yogurt, flaxseed meal, honey, and almond milk until smooth.

Add ice cubes and blend again.

Pour into a glass and relish the cranberry-orange zing.

Cooking Time: Approximately 5 minutes

35. Avocado Berry Bliss Smoothie

Ingredients:

1/2 avocado, peeled and diced

1/2 cup mixed berries (strawberries, blueberries, raspberries)

1/2 cup plain Greek yogurt

1 tablespoon chia seeds

1 tablespoon honey (optional)

1 cup coconut water

Ice cubes

Instructions:

Blend avocado, mixed berries, Greek yogurt, chia seeds, honey, and coconut water until smooth.

Add ice cubes and blend again.

Pour into a glass and savor the avocado-berry bliss.

CONCLUSION

Incorporating smoothies into a diet for colitis can be a beneficial and enjoyable way to support digestive health. By blending nutrient-rich ingredients like fruits, vegetables, and yogurt, individuals with colitis can create easily digestible and soothing beverages that may help alleviate symptoms and provide essential vitamins and minerals.

However, it is important to customize smoothie recipes based on personal tolerance and preferences, and to consult with a healthcare professional for personalized dietary advice. Smoothies can be a flavorful addition to a well-balanced approach to managing colitis and promoting overall well-being.

www.ingramcontent.com/pod-product-compliance
Lightning Source LLC
Chambersburg PA
CBHW070735260726
48660CB00007B/2851